The
Fat
Flush

Journal and Shopping Guide

The Fat Flush

Journal and Shopping Guide

ANN LOUISE GITTLEMAN
M.S., C.N.S.

McGraw-Hill

New York / Chicago / San Francisco / Lisbon / London
Madrid / Mexico City / Milan / New Delhi / San Juan
Seoul / Singapore / Sydney / Toronto

1 2 3 4 5 6 7 8 9 0   DOC/DOC   0 9 8 7 6 5 4 3 2

ISBN 0-07-141497-5

McGraw-Hill books are available at special discounts to use as premiums and sales promotions, or for use in corporate training programs. For more information, please write to the Director of Special Sales, Professional Publishing, McGraw-Hill, Two Penn Plaza, New York, NY 10121-2298. Or contact your local bookstore.

This book is for educational purposes. It is not intended as a substitute for medical advice. Please consult a qualified health care professional for individual health and medical advice. Neither McGraw-Hill nor the author shall have any responsibility for any adverse effects arising directly or indirectly as a result of the information provided in this book.

Throughout this book, trademarked names are used. Rather than put a trademark symbol after every occurrence of a trademarked name, we use names in an editorial fashion only, and to the benefit of the trademark owner, with no intention of infringement of the trademark. Where such designations appear in this book, they have been printed with initial caps.

 This book is printed on recycled, acid-free paper containing a minimum of 50% recycled de-inked paper.

Introduction

Learning to listen to ourselves is a way of learning to love ourselves.

—*Joan Borysenko*

Quite simply, the Fat Flush Plan is designed to renew, recharge, and refresh your body and soul, to allow you to reconnect with yourself.

I know from my own personal experience and from receiving your emails and letters throughout the past 10 years that, for the thousands of men and women who have fully embraced the program, Fat Flush is a rebirth of your physical and mental well-being.

However, as you have no doubt experienced by now, Fat Flush is much more than just a weight loss program. It's a complete lifestyle transformation that makes you feel so good and makes you feel so good about yourself (your clothes start to feel looser, your energy increases, your cravings diminish, and your skin glows like a baby's) that you simply choose *not* to relapse into those old habits which don't support your best self.

Yet, sometimes you may need a gentle nudge, a little reminder to keep you inspired, stay motivated, stay in tune with your body's natural rhythms, or get you back on track. And that's why keeping a journal is such an important component of the Fat Flush experience. This journal provides a safe haven or sanctuary where you don't have to take care of anybody but yourself. It allows you reflective time to discover what's going on inside of you.

For many of you, this journal may be the *only* opportunity where, for 10 to 15 minutes at the end of the day, you get to reflect and be completely honest about yourself in such Fat Flush related areas as your goals for each phase of your journey; what kind of reward you want to treat yourself to when you achieve your goal; what meals, beverages, and snacks you are actually consuming on a daily basis; what supplements you are taking; what your weekly measurements are; what the status is of your health and wellness, your exercise routine, your sleep time; and what you have to say about your reflections and daily acknowledgment.

I'm a firm believer in throwing out the scale—not throwing in the towel—when you don't see your weight budging. While I provide space for you to record your weight, always keep in mind that as you begin to tone up, your size can decrease while your weight may remain the same. Remember that muscle weighs more than fat. The best measurement of success is your tape measure, which is why I want you to measure yourself once a week.

While you're writing, you don't have to fill in every single one of the categories—just the ones that you relate to most. I personally enjoy jotting down my stream-of-consciousness thoughts in the Food for Thought category. One Fat Flusher from Spokane, Washington, told me that she enjoys this category too and discovered that she was better able to identify her food-connected patterns, moods, and emotions by writing about them on a daily basis. She could easily identify her anger and boredom throughout the day, but when she connected her end-of-the-day sweet treats to unresolved stress and fatigue, she viewed this as a major insight. She is now learning to destress after work by taking a late afternoon yoga class so that she doesn't address these emotions by eating cheesecake.

Moreover, the *Fat Flush Journal* helps you keep tabs of all the little steps along the way in your personal Fat Flush journey. As the latest research continues to show, it is those baby-step changes that you make day by day in your eating habits that have the longest-lasting effects. For example, many Fat Flushers use phase 1 for periodic detox and cleansing and follow their regular eating programs for the rest of the time. But, they integrate the Long Life Cocktail and the lemon and water (and flaxseed oil, of course) as part of their "normal" dietary regimens.

This journal can help you to identify the unconscious physical and/or emotional roadblocks to both weight loss and overall health, thus enabling you to fix them and get back in the driver's seat. There's a Chinese proverb I find helpful: "The glory is not in never failing, but in rising each time you fail." Repeating this quote and journaling through the experience should help to take away your guilt and remorse when you deviate from the Fat Flush path. I've included other motivational quotes within the journal so that you can find a bit of daily inspiration each time you write.

Daily journaling can also help to pinpoint where you need to tweak your diet if you have hit a plateau. It can help you to set realistic goals and know when you have achieved them. It can help you get back to your authentic self and regain your personal power.

In addition to the journal pages, I have provided a shopping list to make Fat Flush as convenient as possible on the shopping front. As discussed in *The Fat Flush Cookbook,* the program has evolved and new research has become available. I've expanded the original listings, giving you greater variety and taste satisfaction with additional Fat Flush–friendly foods and seasoning options. Users of the diet will notice that some herbs have moved to an earlier phase; rest assured that this will not affect your weight-loss plan and that these moves are true to Fat Flush principles. Many of these items can be found in your local supermarket or health food store. The categories are organized, as much as possible, by supermarket shopping aisles.

I personally congratulate each and every one of you who are so courageous in striking out to lead a more conscious and balanced life. The time has come for you to start to recognize and acknowledge your own progress in making better diet and lifestyle choices.

Now, let the journaling begin!

The Fat Flush

Journal and Shopping Guide

My Fat Flush Journal

TODAY'S DATE _May 11th_

MY PHASE ____ **GOAL** _130 Lbs Rosie_ _170 lbs Mike_

Lose (67lbs) (80)lbs

By Wedding (50lbs) (50lbs)

MEASUREMENTS	(R)	2/26/04	(M)	2/26/04
• Bust/Chest	50	50	45½	47
• Waist	44	45	51½	52
• Hips	46	48	45	47
• Thighs	25	25½	28	30
• Weight	197	201	250	260

WHY I WANT TO REACH MY GOAL

(R) This is not how I Remember Myself.
I Feel tired, My Skin is Suffering, &
because everything I wear looks sloppy & uncomfortable
I don't want to Shop for Stretchy Clothing anymore
(M) I hate being Fat, I want to Feel better
about Myself & in My Clothing, I want to
have engery & stiama for My Honeymoon.
(B) " * Wedding pictures "

MY PHASE ____ **REWARD** _____

DAY 1

And if not now, when?

—*The Talmud*

TODAY'S DATE _____

MEALS, BEVERAGES, AND SNACKS

• Upon rising _____

• Before breakfast _____

• Breakfast _____

_____

• Midmorning snack _____

• Before lunch _____   _____

• Lunch _____

_____

_____

_____

• Midafternoon snack _____

• 4 P.M. snack _____

• Before dinner _____

• Dinner _____

_____

_____

_____

_____

• Midevening _____

SUPPLEMENTS _____

_____

_____

EXERCISE _____

_____

_____

_____

_____

HEALTH AND WELLNESS NOTES _____

_____

_____

_____

_____

FOOD FOR THOUGHT _____

_____

_____

_____

_____

SLEEP TIME _____

_____

_____

REFLECTIONS _____

_____

_____

_____

_____

DAILY ACKNOWLEDGMENT _____

_____

_____

_____

_____

_____

DAY 2

If you want to see what your thoughts were like yesterday, look at your body today. If you want to see what your body will be like tomorrow, look at your thoughts today.

—*Indian Proverb*

TODAY'S DATE _____

MEALS, BEVERAGES, AND SNACKS

• Upon rising _____

• Before breakfast _____

• Breakfast _____

_____

• Midmorning snack _____

• Before lunch _____

• Lunch _____

_____

_____

_____

• Midafternoon snack _____

• 4 P.M. snack _____

• Before dinner _____

• Dinner _____

_____

_____

_____

_____

• Midevening _____

SUPPLEMENTS _____

_____

_____

EXERCISE _____

_____

_____

_____

_____

HEALTH AND WELLNESS NOTES _____

_____

_____

_____

_____

FOOD FOR THOUGHT _____

_____

_____

_____

_____

SLEEP TIME _____

_____

_____

REFLECTIONS _____

_____

_____

_____

_____

DAILY ACKNOWLEDGMENT _____

_____

_____

_____

_____

_____

DAY 3

I have learned, as a rule of thumb, never to ask whether you can do something. Say, instead, that you are doing it. Then fasten your seat belt. The most remarkable things follow.

—*Julia Cameron*

TODAY'S DATE _____

MEALS, BEVERAGES, AND SNACKS

• Upon rising _____

• Before breakfast _____

• Breakfast _____

_____

• Midmorning snack _____

• Before lunch _____

• Lunch _____

_____

_____

_____

• Midafternoon snack _____

• 4 P.M. snack _____

• Before dinner _____

• Dinner _____

_____

_____

_____

_____

• Midevening _____

SUPPLEMENTS _____

_____

_____

Day 3

EXERCISE _____
_____
_____
_____
_____

HEALTH AND WELLNESS NOTES _____
_____
_____
_____
_____

FOOD FOR THOUGHT _____
_____
_____
_____
_____

SLEEP TIME _____
_____
_____

REFLECTIONS _____
_____
_____
_____
_____

DAILY ACKNOWLEDGMENT _____
_____
_____
_____
_____
_____

DAY 4

Tough times never last; tough people do.

—*Robert Schuller*

TODAY'S DATE _____

MEALS, BEVERAGES, AND SNACKS

• Upon rising _____

• Before breakfast _____

• Breakfast _____

_____

• Midmorning snack _____

• Before lunch _____

• Lunch _____

_____

_____

_____

• Midafternoon snack _____

• 4 P.M. snack _____

• Before dinner _____

• Dinner _____

_____

_____

_____

_____

• Midevening _____

SUPPLEMENTS _____

_____

_____

Day 4

EXERCISE _____

_____

_____

_____

_____

HEALTH AND WELLNESS NOTES _____

_____

_____

_____

_____

FOOD FOR THOUGHT _____

_____

_____

_____

_____

SLEEP TIME _____

_____

_____

REFLECTIONS _____

_____

_____

_____

_____

DAILY ACKNOWLEDGMENT _____

_____

_____

_____

_____

_____

DAY 5

> *I have an everyday religion that works for me. Love yourself first and everything else falls into line.*
>
> —*Lucille Ball*

TODAY'S DATE _____

MEALS, BEVERAGES, AND SNACKS

• Upon rising _____

• Before breakfast _____

• Breakfast _____

_____

• Midmorning snack _____

• Before lunch _____

• Lunch _____

_____

_____

_____

• Midafternoon snack _____

• 4 P.M. snack _____

• Before dinner _____

• Dinner _____

_____

_____

_____

_____

• Midevening _____

SUPPLEMENTS _____

_____

_____

EXERCISE _____

_____

_____

_____

_____

HEALTH AND WELLNESS NOTES _____

_____

_____

_____

_____

FOOD FOR THOUGHT _____

_____

_____

_____

_____

SLEEP TIME _____

_____

_____

REFLECTIONS _____

_____

_____

_____

_____

DAILY ACKNOWLEDGMENT _____

_____

_____

_____

_____

_____

DAY 6

> *There are some things you learn best in calm, and some in storm.*
>
> —*Willa Cather*

TODAY'S DATE _____

MEALS, BEVERAGES, AND SNACKS

• Upon rising _____

• Before breakfast _____

• Breakfast _____

_____

• Midmorning snack _____

• Before lunch _____

• Lunch _____

_____

_____

_____

• Midafternoon snack _____

• 4 P.M. snack _____

• Before dinner _____

• Dinner _____

_____

_____

_____

_____

• Midevening _____

SUPPLEMENTS _____

_____

_____

EXERCISE _____

_____

_____

_____

_____

HEALTH AND WELLNESS NOTES _____

_____

_____

_____

_____

FOOD FOR THOUGHT _____

_____

_____

_____

_____

SLEEP TIME _____

_____

_____

REFLECTIONS _____

_____

_____

_____

_____

DAILY ACKNOWLEDGMENT _____

_____

_____

_____

_____

_____

DAY 7

If we all did the things we are capable of doing, we would literally astound ourselves.

—*Thomas Edison*

TODAY'S DATE _____

MEALS, BEVERAGES, AND SNACKS

• Upon rising _____

• Before breakfast _____

• Breakfast _____

_____

• Midmorning snack _____

• Before lunch _____

• Lunch _____

_____

_____

_____

• Midafternoon snack _____

• 4 P.M. snack _____

• Before dinner _____

• Dinner _____

_____

_____

_____

_____

• Midevening _____

SUPPLEMENTS _____

_____

_____

EXERCISE _____

_____

_____

_____

_____

HEALTH AND WELLNESS NOTES _____

_____

_____

_____

_____

FOOD FOR THOUGHT _____

_____

_____

_____

_____

SLEEP TIME _____

_____

_____

REFLECTIONS _____

_____

_____

_____

_____

DAILY ACKNOWLEDGMENT _____

_____

_____

_____

_____

_____

WEEK 1 PROGRESS

MY THOUGHTS ABOUT THE PAST WEEK: _____

_____

_____

_____

_____

_____

_____

_____

_____

_____

_____

_____

_____

OVER THE PAST WEEK, HERE'S WHAT I'VE NOTICED ABOUT:

• The fit of my clothes _____

_____

_____

• My sleep patterns _____

_____

_____

• My energy level _____

_____

_____

• My skin _____

_____

_____

MEASUREMENTS

- Bust/chest _____
- Waist _____
- Hips _____
- Thighs _____
- Weight _____

MY BIGGEST TEMPTATION _____
_____
_____

MY BEST COMPLIMENT _____
_____
_____

MY PROUDEST MOMENT _____
_____
_____

MY CHALLENGES AND GOALS FOR THE UPCOMING WEEK _____
_____
_____
_____
_____

MY REWARD FOR A WEEK OF PROGRESS _____
_____
_____
_____
_____

DAY 8

Whatever your mind can conceive and believe, it will achieve.

—*Anonymous*

TODAY'S DATE _____

MEALS, BEVERAGES, AND SNACKS

• Upon rising _____

• Before breakfast _____

• Breakfast _____

_____

• Midmorning snack _____

• Before lunch _____

• Lunch _____

_____

_____

_____

• Midafternoon snack _____

• 4 P.M. snack _____

• Before dinner _____

• Dinner _____

_____

_____

_____

_____

• Midevening _____

SUPPLEMENTS _____

_____

_____

EXERCISE _____

_____

_____

_____

_____

HEALTH AND WELLNESS NOTES _____

_____

_____

_____

_____

FOOD FOR THOUGHT _____

_____

_____

_____

_____

SLEEP TIME _____

_____

_____

REFLECTIONS _____

_____

_____

_____

_____

DAILY ACKNOWLEDGMENT _____

_____

_____

_____

_____

DAY 9

All acts of healing are ultimately ourselves healing our Self.
—Ram Dass

TODAY'S DATE _____

MEALS, BEVERAGES, AND SNACKS

• Upon rising _____

• Before breakfast _____

• Breakfast _____

_____

• Midmorning snack _____

• Before lunch _____

• Lunch _____

_____

_____

_____

• Midafternoon snack _____

• 4 P.M. snack _____

• Before dinner _____

• Dinner _____

_____

_____

_____

_____

• Midevening _____

SUPPLEMENTS _____

_____

_____

EXERCISE _____

_____

_____

_____

_____

HEALTH AND WELLNESS NOTES _____

_____

_____

_____

_____

FOOD FOR THOUGHT _____

_____

_____

_____

_____

SLEEP TIME _____

_____

_____

REFLECTIONS _____

_____

_____

_____

_____

DAILY ACKNOWLEDGMENT _____

_____

_____

_____

_____

_____

DAY 10

> *To remain healthy, many must have some goal, some pur-*
> *pose in life that they can respect and be proud to work for.*
>
> —*Hans Selye*

TODAY'S DATE _____

MEALS, BEVERAGES, AND SNACKS

• Upon rising _____

• Before breakfast _____

• Breakfast _____

_____

• Midmorning snack _____

• Before lunch _____

• Lunch _____

_____

_____

_____

• Midafternoon snack _____

• 4 P.M. snack _____

• Before dinner _____

• Dinner _____

_____

_____

_____

_____

• Midevening _____

SUPPLEMENTS _____

_____

_____

EXERCISE _____

_____

_____

_____

_____

HEALTH AND WELLNESS NOTES _____

_____

_____

_____

_____

FOOD FOR THOUGHT _____

_____

_____

_____

_____

SLEEP TIME _____

_____

_____

REFLECTIONS _____

_____

_____

_____

_____

DAILY ACKNOWLEDGMENT _____

_____

_____

_____

_____

DAY 11

Genius is nothing but continued attention.

—Helvetius

TODAY'S DATE _____

MEALS, BEVERAGES, AND SNACKS

• Upon rising _____

• Before breakfast _____

• Breakfast _____

_____

• Midmorning snack _____

• Before lunch _____

• Lunch _____

_____

_____

_____

• Midafternoon snack _____

• 4 P.M. snack _____

• Before dinner _____

• Dinner _____

_____

_____

_____

_____

• Midevening _____

SUPPLEMENTS _____

_____

_____

EXERCISE _____

_____

_____

_____

_____

HEALTH AND WELLNESS NOTES _____

_____

_____

_____

_____

FOOD FOR THOUGHT _____

_____

_____

_____

_____

SLEEP TIME _____

_____

_____

REFLECTIONS _____

_____

_____

_____

_____

DAILY ACKNOWLEDGMENT _____

_____

_____

_____

_____

_____

DAY 12

The quality of a person's life is in direct proportion to their commitment to excellence, regardless of the chosen field or endeavor.

—*Vince Lombardi*

TODAY'S DATE _____

MEALS, BEVERAGES, AND SNACKS

• Upon rising _____

• Before breakfast _____

• Breakfast _____

_____

• Midmorning snack _____

• Before lunch _____

• Lunch _____

_____

_____

_____

• Midafternoon snack _____

• 4 P.M. snack _____

• Before dinner _____

• Dinner _____

_____

_____

_____

_____

• Midevening _____

SUPPLEMENTS _____

_____

_____

EXERCISE _____

_____

_____

_____

_____

HEALTH AND WELLNESS NOTES _____

_____

_____

_____

_____

FOOD FOR THOUGHT _____

_____

_____

_____

_____

SLEEP TIME _____

_____

_____

REFLECTIONS _____

_____

_____

_____

_____

DAILY ACKNOWLEDGMENT _____

_____

_____

_____

_____

_____

DAY 13

All seasons of life are beautiful. Aging is a problem only when you stop liking yourself as a person.

—*Sophia Loren*

TODAY'S DATE _____

MEALS, BEVERAGES, AND SNACKS

• Upon rising _____

• Before breakfast _____

• Breakfast _____

_____

• Midmorning snack _____

• Before lunch _____

• Lunch _____

_____

_____

_____

• Midafternoon snack _____

• 4 P.M. snack _____

• Before dinner _____

• Dinner _____

_____

_____

_____

_____

• Midevening _____

SUPPLEMENTS _____

_____

_____

EXERCISE _____

_____

_____

_____

_____

HEALTH AND WELLNESS NOTES _____

_____

_____

_____

_____

FOOD FOR THOUGHT _____

_____

_____

_____

_____

SLEEP TIME _____

_____

_____

REFLECTIONS _____

_____

_____

_____

_____

DAILY ACKNOWLEDGMENT _____

_____

_____

_____

_____

_____

DAY 14

Many persons have a wrong idea of what constitutes true happiness. It is not attained through self-gratification but through fidelity to a worthy purpose.

—*Helen Keller*

TODAY'S DATE _____

MEALS, BEVERAGES, AND SNACKS

• Upon rising _____

• Before breakfast _____

• Breakfast _____

_____

• Midmorning snack _____

• Before lunch _____

• Lunch _____

_____

_____

_____

• Midafternoon snack _____

• 4 P.M. snack _____

• Before dinner _____

• Dinner _____

_____

_____

_____

_____

• Midevening _____

SUPPLEMENTS _____

_____

_____

EXERCISE _____

_____

_____

_____

_____

HEALTH AND WELLNESS NOTES _____

_____

_____

_____

_____

FOOD FOR THOUGHT _____

_____

_____

_____

_____

SLEEP TIME _____

_____

_____

REFLECTIONS _____

_____

_____

_____

_____

DAILY ACKNOWLEDGMENT _____

_____

_____

_____

_____

_____

WEEK 2 PROGRESS

MY THOUGHTS ABOUT THE PAST WEEK: _____

_____

_____

_____

_____

_____

_____

_____

_____

_____

_____

_____

OVER THE PAST WEEK, HERE'S WHAT I'VE NOTICED ABOUT:

• The fit of my clothes _____

_____

_____

• My sleep patterns _____

_____

_____

• My energy level _____

_____

_____

• My skin _____

_____

_____

MEASUREMENTS

- Bust/chest _____
- Waist _____
- Hips _____
- Thighs _____
- Weight _____

MY BIGGEST TEMPTATION _____

_____

_____

MY BEST COMPLIMENT _____

_____

_____

MY PROUDEST MOMENT _____

_____

_____

MY CHALLENGES AND GOALS FOR THE UPCOMING WEEK _____

_____

_____

_____

_____

_____

MY REWARD FOR A WEEK OF PROGRESS _____

_____

_____

_____

_____

DAY 15

> *One of the things I learned the hard way was that it doesn't pay to get discouraged. Keeping busy and making optimism a way of life can restore your faith in yourself.*
>
> —Lucille Ball

TODAY'S DATE _____

MEALS, BEVERAGES, AND SNACKS

• Upon rising _____

• Before breakfast _____

• Breakfast _____

_____

• Midmorning snack _____

• Before lunch _____

• Lunch _____

_____

_____

_____

• Midafternoon snack _____

• 4 P.M. snack _____

• Before dinner _____

• Dinner _____

_____

_____

_____

_____

• Midevening _____

SUPPLEMENTS _____

_____

_____

EXERCISE _____

_____

_____

_____

_____

HEALTH AND WELLNESS NOTES _____

_____

_____

_____

_____

FOOD FOR THOUGHT _____

_____

_____

_____

_____

SLEEP TIME _____

_____

_____

REFLECTIONS _____

_____

_____

_____

_____

DAILY ACKNOWLEDGMENT _____

_____

_____

_____

_____

DAY 16

The way I see it, if you want the rainbow, you gotta put up with the rain.

—*Dolly Parton*

TODAY'S DATE _____

MEALS, BEVERAGES, AND SNACKS

• Upon rising _____

• Before breakfast _____

• Breakfast _____

_____

• Midmorning snack _____

• Before lunch _____

• Lunch _____

_____

_____

_____

• Midafternoon snack _____

• 4 P.M. snack _____

• Before dinner _____

• Dinner _____

_____

_____

_____

_____

• Midevening _____

SUPPLEMENTS _____

_____

_____

EXERCISE _____

_____

_____

_____

_____

HEALTH AND WELLNESS NOTES _____

_____

_____

_____

_____

FOOD FOR THOUGHT _____

_____

_____

_____

_____

SLEEP TIME _____

_____

_____

REFLECTIONS _____

_____

_____

_____

_____

DAILY ACKNOWLEDGMENT _____

_____

_____

_____

_____

_____

DAY 17

Whatever you can do, or dream you can, begin it. Boldness has genius, power and magic in it.

—*Goethe*

TODAY'S DATE _____

MEALS, BEVERAGES, AND SNACKS

• Upon rising _____

• Before breakfast _____

• Breakfast _____

_____

• Midmorning snack _____

• Before lunch _____

• Lunch _____

_____

_____

_____

• Midafternoon snack _____

• 4 P.M. snack _____

• Before dinner _____

• Dinner _____

_____

_____

_____

_____

• Midevening _____

SUPPLEMENTS _____

_____

_____

EXERCISE _____

_____

_____

_____

_____

HEALTH AND WELLNESS NOTES _____

_____

_____

_____

_____

FOOD FOR THOUGHT _____

_____

_____

_____

_____

SLEEP TIME _____

_____

_____

REFLECTIONS _____

_____

_____

_____

_____

DAILY ACKNOWLEDGMENT _____

_____

_____

_____

_____

DAY 18

Ladies—your kitchen is the laboratory of life—you are the kitchen chemist—be sure you know your business.

—Dr. Hazel Parcells

TODAY'S DATE _____

MEALS, BEVERAGES, AND SNACKS

• Upon rising _____

• Before breakfast _____

• Breakfast _____

_____

• Midmorning snack _____

• Before lunch _____

• Lunch _____

_____

_____

_____

• Midafternoon snack _____

• 4 P.M. snack _____

• Before dinner _____

• Dinner _____

_____

_____

_____

_____

• Midevening _____

SUPPLEMENTS _____

_____

_____

EXERCISE _____

_____

_____

_____

_____

HEALTH AND WELLNESS NOTES _____

_____

_____

_____

_____

FOOD FOR THOUGHT _____

_____

_____

_____

_____

SLEEP TIME _____

_____

_____

REFLECTIONS _____

_____

_____

_____

_____

DAILY ACKNOWLEDGMENT _____

_____

_____

_____

_____

_____

DAY 19

Just pray for a thick skin and a tender heart.

—*Ruth Bell Graham*

TODAY'S DATE _____

MEALS, BEVERAGES, AND SNACKS

• Upon rising _____

• Before breakfast _____

• Breakfast _____

_____

• Midmorning snack _____

• Before lunch _____

• Lunch _____

_____

_____

_____

• Midafternoon snack _____

• 4 P.M. snack _____

• Before dinner _____

• Dinner _____

_____

_____

_____

_____

• Midevening _____

SUPPLEMENTS _____

_____

_____

Day 19

EXERCISE _____

_____

_____

_____

_____

HEALTH AND WELLNESS NOTES _____

_____

_____

_____

_____

FOOD FOR THOUGHT _____

_____

_____

_____

_____

SLEEP TIME _____

_____

_____

REFLECTIONS _____

_____

_____

_____

_____

DAILY ACKNOWLEDGMENT _____

_____

_____

_____

_____

_____

DAY 20

If you want to break a habit—you must do it immediately and flamboyantly.

—*William James*

TODAY'S DATE _____

MEALS, BEVERAGES, AND SNACKS

• Upon rising _____

• Before breakfast _____

• Breakfast _____

_____

• Midmorning snack _____

• Before lunch _____

• Lunch _____

_____

_____

_____

• Midafternoon snack _____

• 4 P.M. snack _____

• Before dinner _____

• Dinner _____

_____

_____

_____

_____

• Midevening _____

SUPPLEMENTS _____

_____

_____

EXERCISE _____

_____

_____

_____

_____

HEALTH AND WELLNESS NOTES _____

_____

_____

_____

_____

FOOD FOR THOUGHT _____

_____

_____

_____

_____

SLEEP TIME _____

_____

_____

REFLECTIONS _____

_____

_____

_____

_____

DAILY ACKNOWLEDGMENT _____

_____

_____

_____

_____

DAY 21

A cheerful heart hath a continual feast.

—*Proverbs 15:15*

TODAY'S DATE _____

MEALS, BEVERAGES, AND SNACKS

• Upon rising _____

• Before breakfast _____

• Breakfast _____

_____

• Midmorning snack _____

• Before lunch _____

• Lunch _____

_____

_____

_____

• Midafternoon snack _____

• 4 P.M. snack _____

• Before dinner _____

• Dinner _____

_____

_____

_____

_____

• Midevening _____

SUPPLEMENTS _____

_____

_____

EXERCISE _____

_____

_____

_____

_____

HEALTH AND WELLNESS NOTES _____

_____

_____

_____

_____

FOOD FOR THOUGHT _____

_____

_____

_____

_____

SLEEP TIME _____

_____

_____

REFLECTIONS _____

_____

_____

_____

_____

DAILY ACKNOWLEDGMENT _____

_____

_____

_____

_____

_____

WEEK 3 PROGRESS

MY THOUGHTS ABOUT THE PAST WEEK: _____

_____

_____

_____

_____

_____

_____

_____

_____

_____

_____

_____

OVER THE PAST WEEK, HERE'S WHAT I'VE NOTICED ABOUT:

• The fit of my clothes _____

_____

_____

• My sleep patterns _____

_____

_____

• My energy level _____

_____

_____

• My skin _____

_____

_____

MEASUREMENTS

- Bust/chest _____
- Waist _____
- Hips _____
- Thighs _____
- Weight _____

MY BIGGEST TEMPTATION _____

_____

_____

MY BEST COMPLIMENT _____

_____

_____

MY PROUDEST MOMENT _____

_____

_____

MY CHALLENGES AND GOALS FOR THE UPCOMING WEEK _____

_____

_____

_____

_____

_____

MY REWARD FOR A WEEK OF PROGRESS _____

_____

_____

_____

_____

DAY 22

Tell me what you eat and I will tell you what you are.
—Athelme Brillat-Savarin

TODAY'S DATE _____

MEALS, BEVERAGES, AND SNACKS

• Upon rising _____

• Before breakfast _____

• Breakfast _____

_____

• Midmorning snack _____

• Before lunch _____

• Lunch _____

_____

_____

_____

• Midafternoon snack _____

• 4 P.M. snack _____

• Before dinner _____

• Dinner _____

_____

_____

_____

_____

• Midevening _____

SUPPLEMENTS _____

_____

_____

EXERCISE _____

_____

_____

_____

_____

HEALTH AND WELLNESS NOTES _____

_____

_____

_____

_____

FOOD FOR THOUGHT _____

_____

_____

_____

_____

SLEEP TIME _____

_____

_____

REFLECTIONS _____

_____

_____

_____

_____

DAILY ACKNOWLEDGMENT _____

_____

_____

_____

_____

DAY 23

We're always the same age inside.

—*Gertrude Stein*

TODAY'S DATE _____

MEALS, BEVERAGES, AND SNACKS

• **Upon rising** _____

• **Before breakfast** _____

• **Breakfast** _____

_____

• **Midmorning snack** _____

• **Before lunch** _____

• **Lunch** _____

_____

_____

_____

• **Midafternoon snack** _____

• **4 P.M. snack** _____

• **Before dinner** _____

• **Dinner** _____

_____

_____

_____

_____

• **Midevening** _____

SUPPLEMENTS _____

_____

_____

EXERCISE _____

_____

_____

_____

_____

HEALTH AND WELLNESS NOTES _____

_____

_____

_____

_____

FOOD FOR THOUGHT _____

_____

_____

_____

_____

SLEEP TIME _____

_____

_____

REFLECTIONS _____

_____

_____

_____

_____

DAILY ACKNOWLEDGMENT _____

_____

_____

_____

_____

_____

DAY 24

Fitness isn't a job or obligation, it's the natural result of making good, positive lifestyle choices every day.

—Joanie Greggains

TODAY'S DATE _____

MEALS, BEVERAGES, AND SNACKS

• Upon rising _____

• Before breakfast _____

• Breakfast _____

_____

• Midmorning snack _____

• Before lunch _____

• Lunch _____

_____

_____

_____

• Midafternoon snack _____

• 4 P.M. snack _____

• Before dinner _____

• Dinner _____

_____

_____

_____

_____

• Midevening _____

SUPPLEMENTS _____

_____

_____

EXERCISE _____

_____

_____

_____

_____

HEALTH AND WELLNESS NOTES _____

_____

_____

_____

_____

FOOD FOR THOUGHT _____

_____

_____

_____

_____

SLEEP TIME _____

_____

_____

REFLECTIONS _____

_____

_____

_____

_____

DAILY ACKNOWLEDGMENT _____

_____

_____

_____

_____

_____

DAY 25

Man's main task in life is to give birth to himself.

—*Erich Fromm*

TODAY'S DATE _____

MEALS, BEVERAGES, AND SNACKS

• Upon rising _____

• Before breakfast _____

• Breakfast _____

_____

• Midmorning snack _____

• Before lunch _____

• Lunch _____

_____

_____

_____

• Midafternoon snack _____

• 4 P.M. snack _____

• Before dinner _____

• Dinner _____

_____

_____

_____

_____

• Midevening _____

SUPPLEMENTS _____

_____

_____

EXERCISE _____

_____

_____

_____

_____

HEALTH AND WELLNESS NOTES _____

_____

_____

_____

_____

FOOD FOR THOUGHT _____

_____

_____

_____

_____

SLEEP TIME _____

_____

_____

REFLECTIONS _____

_____

_____

_____

_____

DAILY ACKNOWLEDGMENT _____

_____

_____

_____

_____

_____

DAY 26

Why separate your spiritual life and your practical life? To an integral being, there is no such distinction.

—*Lao Tzu*

TODAY'S DATE _____

MEALS, BEVERAGES, AND SNACKS

• Upon rising _____

• Before breakfast _____

• Breakfast _____

_____

• Midmorning snack _____

• Before lunch _____

• Lunch _____

_____

_____

_____

• Midafternoon snack _____

• 4 P.M. snack _____

• Before dinner _____

• Dinner _____

_____

_____

_____

_____

• Midevening _____

SUPPLEMENTS _____

_____

_____

EXERCISE _____

_____

_____

_____

_____

HEALTH AND WELLNESS NOTES _____

_____

_____

_____

_____

FOOD FOR THOUGHT _____

_____

_____

_____

_____

SLEEP TIME _____

_____

_____

REFLECTIONS _____

_____

_____

_____

_____

DAILY ACKNOWLEDGMENT _____

_____

_____

_____

_____

_____

DAY 27

The hero is the man who is immovably centered.
—Ralph Waldo Emerson

TODAY'S DATE _____

MEALS, BEVERAGES, AND SNACKS

• Upon rising _____

• Before breakfast _____

• Breakfast _____

_____

• Midmorning snack _____

• Before lunch _____

• Lunch _____

_____

_____

_____

• Midafternoon snack _____

• 4 P.M. snack _____

• Before dinner _____

• Dinner _____

_____

_____

_____

_____

• Midevening _____

SUPPLEMENTS _____

_____

_____

Day 27

EXERCISE _____

_____

_____

_____

_____

HEALTH AND WELLNESS NOTES _____

_____

_____

_____

_____

FOOD FOR THOUGHT _____

_____

_____

_____

_____

SLEEP TIME _____

_____

_____

REFLECTIONS _____

_____

_____

_____

_____

DAILY ACKNOWLEDGMENT _____

_____

_____

_____

_____

_____

DAY 28

You must trust that small voice inside you which tells you exactly what to say, what to decide. Your intuition is your instrument.

—*Ingmar Bergman*

TODAY'S DATE _____

MEALS, BEVERAGES, AND SNACKS

• Upon rising _____

• Before breakfast _____

• Breakfast _____

_____

• Midmorning snack _____

• Before lunch _____

• Lunch _____

_____

_____

_____

• Midafternoon snack _____

• 4 P.M. snack _____

• Before dinner _____

• Dinner _____

_____

_____

_____

_____

• Midevening _____

SUPPLEMENTS _____

_____

_____

EXERCISE _____

_____

_____

_____

_____

HEALTH AND WELLNESS NOTES _____

_____

_____

_____

_____

FOOD FOR THOUGHT _____

_____

_____

_____

_____

SLEEP TIME _____

_____

_____

REFLECTIONS _____

_____

_____

_____

_____

DAILY ACKNOWLEDGMENT _____

_____

_____

_____

_____

_____

WEEK 4 PROGRESS

MY THOUGHTS ABOUT THE PAST WEEK: _____

_____

_____

_____

_____

_____

_____

_____

_____

_____

_____

_____

OVER THE PAST WEEK, HERE'S WHAT I'VE NOTICED ABOUT:

• The fit of my clothes _____

_____

_____

• My sleep patterns _____

_____

_____

• My energy level _____

_____

_____

• My skin _____

_____

_____

MEASUREMENTS

- Bust/chest _____
- Waist _____
- Hips _____
- Thighs _____
- Weight _____

MY BIGGEST TEMPTATION _____
_____
_____

MY BEST COMPLIMENT _____
_____
_____

MY PROUDEST MOMENT _____
_____
_____

MY CHALLENGES AND GOALS FOR THE UPCOMING WEEK _____
_____
_____
_____
_____
_____

MY REWARD FOR A WEEK OF PROGRESS _____
_____
_____
_____
_____

DAY 29

In play we reveal what kind of people we are.

—Ovid

TODAY'S DATE _____

MEALS, BEVERAGES, AND SNACKS

• Upon rising _____

• Before breakfast _____

• Breakfast _____

_____

• Midmorning snack _____

• Before lunch _____

• Lunch _____

_____

_____

_____

• Midafternoon snack _____

• 4 P.M. snack _____

• Before dinner _____

• Dinner _____

_____

_____

_____

_____

• Midevening _____

SUPPLEMENTS _____

_____

_____

EXERCISE _____

_____

_____

_____

_____

HEALTH AND WELLNESS NOTES _____

_____

_____

_____

_____

FOOD FOR THOUGHT _____

_____

_____

_____

_____

SLEEP TIME _____

_____

_____

REFLECTIONS _____

_____

_____

_____

DAILY ACKNOWLEDGMENT _____

_____

_____

_____

_____

DAY 30

Life is like playing a violin solo in public and learning the instrument as one goes on.

—Samuel Butler

TODAY'S DATE _____

MEALS, BEVERAGES, AND SNACKS

• Upon rising _____

• Before breakfast _____

• Breakfast _____

_____

• Midmorning snack _____

• Before lunch _____

• Lunch _____

_____

_____

_____

• Midafternoon snack _____

• 4 P.M. snack _____

• Before dinner _____

• Dinner _____

_____

_____

_____

_____

• Midevening _____

SUPPLEMENTS _____

_____

_____

EXERCISE _____

_____

_____

_____

_____

HEALTH AND WELLNESS NOTES _____

_____

_____

_____

_____

FOOD FOR THOUGHT _____

_____

_____

_____

_____

SLEEP TIME _____

_____

_____

REFLECTIONS _____

_____

_____

_____

_____

DAILY ACKNOWLEDGMENT _____

_____

_____

_____

_____

_____

DAY 31

Healing is the intuitive art of wooing nature.

—W.H. Auden

TODAY'S DATE _____

MEALS, BEVERAGES, AND SNACKS

• **Upon rising** _____

• **Before breakfast** _____

• **Breakfast** _____

_____

• **Midmorning snack** _____

• **Before lunch** _____

• **Lunch** _____

_____

_____

_____

• **Midafternoon snack** _____

• **4 P.M. snack** _____

• **Before dinner** _____

• **Dinner** _____

_____

_____

_____

_____

• **Midevening** _____

SUPPLEMENTS _____

_____

_____

EXERCISE _____

_____

_____

_____

_____

HEALTH AND WELLNESS NOTES _____

_____

_____

_____

_____

FOOD FOR THOUGHT _____

_____

_____

_____

_____

SLEEP TIME _____

_____

_____

REFLECTIONS _____

_____

_____

_____

_____

DAILY ACKNOWLEDGMENT _____

_____

_____

_____

_____

_____

DAY 32

Life is not a matter of extent, but of content.

—Stephen S. Wise

TODAY'S DATE _____

MEALS, BEVERAGES, AND SNACKS

• Upon rising _____

• Before breakfast _____

• Breakfast _____

_____

• Midmorning snack _____

• Before lunch _____

• Lunch _____

_____

_____

_____

• Midafternoon snack _____

• 4 P.M. snack _____

• Before dinner _____

• Dinner _____

_____

_____

_____

_____

• Midevening _____

SUPPLEMENTS _____

_____

_____

EXERCISE _____
_____
_____
_____
_____
_____

HEALTH AND WELLNESS NOTES _____
_____
_____
_____
_____

FOOD FOR THOUGHT _____
_____
_____
_____
_____

SLEEP TIME _____
_____
_____

REFLECTIONS _____
_____
_____
_____
_____

DAILY ACKNOWLEDGMENT _____
_____
_____
_____
_____
_____

DAY 33

Flops are a part of life's menu and I've never been a girl to miss out on any of the courses.

—*Rosalind Russell*

TODAY'S DATE _____

MEALS, BEVERAGES, AND SNACKS

• Upon rising _____

• Before breakfast _____

• Breakfast _____

_____

• Midmorning snack _____

• Before lunch _____

• Lunch _____

_____

_____

_____

• Midafternoon snack _____

• 4 P.M. snack _____

• Before dinner _____

• Dinner _____

_____

_____

_____

_____

• Midevening _____

SUPPLEMENTS _____

_____

_____

EXERCISE _____

_____

_____

_____

_____

HEALTH AND WELLNESS NOTES _____

_____

_____

_____

_____

FOOD FOR THOUGHT _____

_____

_____

_____

_____

SLEEP TIME _____

_____

_____

REFLECTIONS _____

_____

_____

_____

DAILY ACKNOWLEDGMENT _____

_____

_____

_____

_____

DAY 34

> *The great thing about getting older is that you don't lose all the other ages you've been.*
>
> —Madeleine L'Engle

TODAY'S DATE _____

MEALS, BEVERAGES, AND SNACKS

• Upon rising _____

• Before breakfast _____

• Breakfast _____

_____

• Midmorning snack _____

• Before lunch _____

• Lunch _____

_____

_____

_____

• Midafternoon snack _____

• 4 P.M. snack _____

• Before dinner _____

• Dinner _____

_____

_____

_____

_____

• Midevening _____

SUPPLEMENTS _____

_____

_____

EXERCISE _____

_____

_____

_____

_____

HEALTH AND WELLNESS NOTES _____

_____

_____

_____

_____

FOOD FOR THOUGHT _____

_____

_____

_____

_____

SLEEP TIME _____

_____

_____

REFLECTIONS _____

_____

_____

_____

DAILY ACKNOWLEDGMENT _____

_____

_____

_____

_____

_____

DAY 35

We need love in order to live happily as much as we need oxygen in order to live at all.

—*Marianne Williamson*

TODAY'S DATE _____

MEALS, BEVERAGES, AND SNACKS

• Upon rising _____

• Before breakfast _____

• Breakfast _____

_____

• Midmorning snack _____

• Before lunch _____

• Lunch _____

_____

_____

_____

• Midafternoon snack _____

• 4 P.M. snack _____

• Before dinner _____

• Dinner _____

_____

_____

_____

_____

• Midevening _____

SUPPLEMENTS _____

_____

_____

EXERCISE _____

_____

_____

_____

_____

_____

HEALTH AND WELLNESS NOTES _____

_____

_____

_____

_____

FOOD FOR THOUGHT _____

_____

_____

_____

_____

SLEEP TIME _____

_____

_____

REFLECTIONS _____

_____

_____

_____

_____

DAILY ACKNOWLEDGMENT _____

_____

_____

_____

_____

_____

WEEK 5 PROGRESS

MY THOUGHTS ABOUT THE PAST WEEK: _____

_____

_____

_____

_____

_____

_____

_____

_____

_____

_____

_____

OVER THE PAST WEEK, HERE'S WHAT I'VE NOTICED ABOUT:

• The fit of my clothes _____

_____

_____

• My sleep patterns _____

_____

_____

• My energy level _____

_____

_____

• My skin _____

_____

_____

MEASUREMENTS

- Bust/chest _____
- Waist _____
- Hips _____
- Thighs _____
- Weight _____

MY BIGGEST TEMPTATION _____

_____

_____

MY BEST COMPLIMENT _____

_____

_____

MY PROUDEST MOMENT _____

_____

_____

MY CHALLENGES AND GOALS FOR THE UPCOMING WEEK _____

_____

_____

_____

_____

_____

MY REWARD FOR A WEEK OF PROGRESS _____

_____

_____

_____

_____

DAY 36

I may not know the key to success, but the key to failure is trying to please everybody.

—*Bill Cosby*

TODAY'S DATE _____

MEALS, BEVERAGES, AND SNACKS

• Upon rising _____

• Before breakfast _____

• Breakfast _____

_____

• Midmorning snack _____

• Before lunch _____

• Lunch _____

_____

_____

_____

• Midafternoon snack _____

• 4 P.M. snack _____

• Before dinner _____

• Dinner _____

_____

_____

_____

_____

• Midevening _____

SUPPLEMENTS _____

_____

_____

EXERCISE _____

_____

_____

_____

_____

HEALTH AND WELLNESS NOTES _____

_____

_____

_____

_____

FOOD FOR THOUGHT _____

_____

_____

_____

_____

SLEEP TIME _____

_____

_____

REFLECTIONS _____

_____

_____

_____

_____

DAILY ACKNOWLEDGMENT _____

_____

_____

_____

_____

_____

DAY 37

Success is never a destination—it's a journey.

—Satenig St. Marie

TODAY'S DATE _____

MEALS, BEVERAGES, AND SNACKS

• **Upon rising** _____

• **Before breakfast** _____

• **Breakfast** _____

_____

• **Midmorning snack** _____

• **Before lunch** _____

• **Lunch** _____

_____

_____

_____

• **Midafternoon snack** _____

• **4 P.M. snack** _____

• **Before dinner** _____

• **Dinner** _____

_____

_____

_____

_____

• **Midevening** _____

SUPPLEMENTS _____

_____

_____

EXERCISE _____

_____

_____

_____

_____

HEALTH AND WELLNESS NOTES _____

_____

_____

_____

_____

FOOD FOR THOUGHT _____

_____

_____

_____

_____

SLEEP TIME _____

_____

_____

REFLECTIONS _____

_____

_____

_____

_____

DAILY ACKNOWLEDGMENT _____

_____

_____

_____

_____

DAY 38

To accomplish great things, you must not only act, but also dream; not only plan, but also believe.

—Anonymous

TODAY'S DATE _____

MEALS, BEVERAGES, AND SNACKS

• Upon rising _____

• Before breakfast _____

• Breakfast _____

_____

• Midmorning snack _____

• Before lunch _____

• Lunch _____

_____

_____

_____

• Midafternoon snack _____

• 4 P.M. snack _____

• Before dinner _____

• Dinner _____

_____

_____

_____

_____

• Midevening _____

SUPPLEMENTS _____

_____

_____

EXERCISE _____

_____

_____

_____

_____

HEALTH AND WELLNESS NOTES _____

_____

_____

_____

_____

FOOD FOR THOUGHT _____

_____

_____

_____

_____

SLEEP TIME _____

_____

_____

REFLECTIONS _____

_____

_____

_____

_____

DAILY ACKNOWLEDGMENT _____

_____

_____

_____

_____

_____

DAY 39

Seek not to find out who you are, seek to determine who you want to be.

—*Neal D. Walsch*

TODAY'S DATE _____

MEALS, BEVERAGES, AND SNACKS

• Upon rising _____

• Before breakfast _____

• Breakfast _____

_____

• Midmorning snack _____

• Before lunch _____

• Lunch _____

_____

_____

_____

• Midafternoon snack _____

• 4 P.M. snack _____

• Before dinner _____

• Dinner _____

_____

_____

_____

_____

• Midevening _____

SUPPLEMENTS _____

_____

_____

EXERCISE _____

_____

_____

_____

_____

HEALTH AND WELLNESS NOTES _____

_____

_____

_____

_____

FOOD FOR THOUGHT _____

_____

_____

_____

_____

SLEEP TIME _____

_____

_____

REFLECTIONS _____

_____

_____

_____

_____

DAILY ACKNOWLEDGMENT _____

_____

_____

_____

_____

_____

DAY 40

Nothing in life is to be feared. It is only to be understood.
—Marie Curie

TODAY'S DATE _____

MEALS, BEVERAGES, AND SNACKS

• Upon rising _____

• Before breakfast _____

• Breakfast _____

_____

• Midmorning snack _____

• Before lunch _____

• Lunch _____

_____

_____

_____

• Midafternoon snack _____

• 4 P.M. snack _____

• Before dinner _____

• Dinner _____

_____

_____

_____

_____

• Midevening _____

SUPPLEMENTS _____

_____

_____

EXERCISE _____

_____

_____

_____

_____

HEALTH AND WELLNESS NOTES _____

_____

_____

_____

_____

FOOD FOR THOUGHT _____

_____

_____

_____

_____

SLEEP TIME _____

_____

_____

REFLECTIONS _____

_____

_____

_____

DAILY ACKNOWLEDGMENT _____

_____

_____

_____

_____

DAY 41

What lies behind us and what lies before us are tiny matters compared to what lies within us.

—*Ralph Waldo Emerson*

TODAY'S DATE _____

MEALS, BEVERAGES, AND SNACKS

• Upon rising _____

• Before breakfast _____

• Breakfast _____

_____

• Midmorning snack _____

• Before lunch _____

• Lunch _____

_____

_____

_____

• Midafternoon snack _____

• 4 P.M. snack _____

• Before dinner _____

• Dinner _____

_____

_____

_____

_____

• Midevening _____

SUPPLEMENTS _____

_____

_____

EXERCISE _____

_____

_____

_____

_____

HEALTH AND WELLNESS NOTES _____

_____

_____

_____

_____

FOOD FOR THOUGHT _____

_____

_____

_____

_____

SLEEP TIME _____

_____

REFLECTIONS _____

_____

_____

_____

DAILY ACKNOWLEDGMENT _____

_____

_____

_____

_____

_____

DAY 42

The body is a sacred garment . . . and should be treated with honor.

—Martha Graham

TODAY'S DATE _____

MEALS, BEVERAGES, AND SNACKS

• Upon rising _____

• Before breakfast _____

• Breakfast _____

_____

• Midmorning snack _____

• Before lunch _____

• Lunch _____

_____

_____

_____

• Midafternoon snack _____

• 4 P.M. snack _____

• Before dinner _____

• Dinner _____

_____

_____

_____

_____

• Midevening _____

SUPPLEMENTS _____

_____

_____

EXERCISE _____

_____

_____

_____

_____

HEALTH AND WELLNESS NOTES _____

_____

_____

_____

_____

FOOD FOR THOUGHT _____

_____

_____

_____

_____

SLEEP TIME _____

_____

_____

REFLECTIONS _____

_____

_____

_____

_____

DAILY ACKNOWLEDGMENT _____

_____

_____

_____

_____

_____

WEEK 6 PROGRESS

MY THOUGHTS ABOUT THE PAST WEEK: _____

_____

_____

_____

_____

_____

_____

_____

_____

_____

_____

_____

OVER THE PAST WEEK, HERE'S WHAT I'VE NOTICED ABOUT:

• The fit of my clothes _____

_____

_____

• My sleep patterns _____

_____

_____

• My energy level _____

_____

_____

• My skin _____

_____

_____

MEASUREMENTS

- Bust/chest _____
- Waist _____
- Hips _____
- Thighs _____
- Weight _____

MY BIGGEST TEMPTATION _____

_____

_____

MY BEST COMPLIMENT _____

_____

_____

MY PROUDEST MOMENT _____

_____

_____

MY CHALLENGES AND GOALS FOR THE UPCOMING WEEK _____

_____

_____

_____

_____

_____

MY REWARD FOR A WEEK OF PROGRESS _____

_____

_____

_____

_____

My Fat Flush Shopping List

Many of the foods on the shopping list can be purchased at your local health food store; whereas others are available in supermarkets. Naturally, organic produce (vegetables and fruit) is preferable (not only are they tastier and fresher, but they do not have all those nasty pesticides, fungicides, and heavy metals your liver has to break down). For this reason, I am providing the names of some of the easier-to-obtain brands in parentheses. But, please check even the brand names list yourself because formulations and therefore ingredients can change periodically. Most items are readily available throughout the country in either health food stores or supermarkets. For others that are not as readily available, I provided a telephone number and Web address for you to get further information.

Let's start shopping!

PHASE 1:
THE TWO-WEEK FAT FLUSH

Eggs

- Eggs Preferable: omega-3–enriched (Gold Circle Farms, The Country Hen, Eggland's Best, Born 3, Pilgrim's Pride EggsPlus)

Protein: Fish

Fresh

- Bass
- Cod
- Grouper
- Haddock

- Halibut
- Mackerel
- Mahimahi
- Orange roughy
- Perch
- Pike
- Pollock
- Salmon
- Sardines
- Snapper
- Sole
- Squid
- Trout
- Tuna
- Whitefish

Canned
- Crabmeat (Featherweight, Seasons, Lillie, Three Star)
- Mackerel
- Salmon
- Sardines
- Tuna

Protein: Shellfish

- Crab
- Lobster
- Scallops
- Shrimp

Protein: Poultry

- White meat of skinned turkey and chicken, either fresh, frozen, or ground (preferably free-range and hormone-free, such as Foster Farms, Harmony Farms, Shelton Farms, and Young Farms)

Protein: Meats

Beef
Slanker's Grass-Fed Meats in Powderly, Texas, at 1-866-SLANKER or 1-903-732-4653 has delicious grass-fed, pasture finished beef. Ask for more information or visit www.texasgrassfedbeef.com.

- Brisket
- Chuck
- Eye of round
- Flank
- London broil
- Round
- Rump
- Sirloin

Lamb

- Leg
- Loin
- Rib

Veal

- Loin
- Rib
- Shoulder

Other Meats

- Bison (buffalo)
- Elk
- Ostrich
- Venison

Vegetables

- Alfalfa sprouts
- Artichoke hearts
- Arugula
- Asparagus
- Bell peppers, red, green, and orange
- Bamboo shoots
- Broccoli
- Brussels sprouts
- Burdock
- Cabbage
- Carrots
- Cauliflower
- Celery
- Chinese cabbage
- Chives
- Collard greens

- Cucumbers
- Daikon
- Eggplant
- Endive
- Escarole
- Green beans
- Hearts of palm
- Jicama
- Kale
- Loose-leaf lettuce, red or green
- Mung bean sprouts
- Mushrooms
- Mustard greens
- Okra
- Olives
- Onions
- Parsley
- Radicchio
- Radishes
- Rhubarb
- Romaine lettuce
- Snow peas
- Spaghetti squash
- Spinach
- Tomatillos
- Tomatoes
  (Tomato products—check a complete list of Muir Glen Organic Products at www.muirglen.com)
  - Muir Glen No Salt Added Diced Tomatoes
  - Muir Glen No Salt Added Tomato Sauce
  - Muir Glen Pizza Sauce
  - Muir Glen Tomato Paste
  - Muir Glen Tomato Purée
  - Muir Glen Whole Peeled Tomatoes
- Water chestnuts
- Watercress
- Yellow squash
- Zucchini

Fruits

- Apples
- Berries (blueberries, blackberries, and raspberries)

- Cherries
- Cranberries (available seasonally)
- Grapefruit
- Lemons (fresh is best, although Santa Cruz Organic 100% Lemon Juice Not from Concentrate will do)
- Limes (fresh is best, although Santa Cruz Organic 100% Lime Juice Not from Concentrate will do)
- Nectarines
- Oranges
- Peaches
- Pears
- Plums
- Pomegranates (available seasonally)
- Strawberries

Herbs, Spices, and All Accompaniments

- Anise
- Apple cider vinegar (Bragg's organic apple cider vinegar is the best I know of, and the nonirradiated herbs and spices from Frontier Herbs and The Spice Hunter are also highly recommended)
- Bay leaves
- Cayenne
- Cinnamon
- Cloves
- Coriander
- Cream of tartar
- Cumin
- Dill (fresh or dried)
- Dried mustard
- Fennel (fresh or garlic)
- Flaxseeds (whole brown or golden yellow flaxseeds in bulk to be ground daily as needed in a coffee grinder, blender, or food processor on the fine setting)
- Garlic (fresh or garlic powder)
- Ginger (fresh or dried)
- Jalapeños (fresh or in cans or jars)
- Onion powder
- Turmeric

Oil

- Cooking Sprays: nonstick cooking sprays made primarily from olive oil

- Oil: high-lignan flaxseed oil (Fat Flushers seem to prefer Health from the Sun, Omega, Flora, and Spectrum)

Low-Sodium or No-Salt-Added Cooking Broths

- Beef
- Chicken
- Fish
- Vegetable (Shelton's, Health Valley, Hain's, and Perfect Addition)

Juices and Other Drinks

- Bottled water (purified, ozonated, ultraviolet-treated, microfiltered, or electrolyte-enhanced)
- Dandelion root tea (Available in most health food stores or through Uni Key at 1-800-888-4353 or visit *www.unikeyhealth .com*)
- Herbal coffee substitute: naturally caffeine-free herbal coffee blended from herbs, grains, fruits, and nuts. (Available from Teeccino at 1-800-498-3434 or 1-800-888-4353; or visit *www. teeccino.com*. Teeccino is brewed like regular coffee and comes in seven flavors: Java, Original, Hazelnut, Vanilla Nut, Amaretto, Mocha, and Chocolate Mint. The lowest-carb flavors are Java, Vanilla Nut, and Hazelnut at 3 grams of carb per serving and Mocha at 4 grams)
- Unsweetened cranberry juice (no sugar, artificial sweeteners, other juices, or corn syrup added; Knudsen's, Trader Joe's, Mountain Sun)
- Unsweetened cranberry juice concentrate made only from straight cranberry (Knudsen's, Tree of Life)
- Unsweetened pomegranate juice (Knudsen's)

Advanced Health Products

Protein Sources

- Protein powders: lactose-free, no-sugar-added, no artificial sweeteners (no aspartame, no acesulfame K, no sucralose or Splenda) no crystalline fructose and only Stevia-sweetened 100% whey protein (note that formulations can change)
- Tempeh
- Tofu (Mori-Nu, White Wave)

Long Life Cocktail
- Ground flaxseeds (FibroFlax or other Certified Organic Milled Flaxseeds)
- Powdered psyllium husks (Yerba Prima or other health food bulk brands)

Sweeteners
- Herbal sweetener (Stevia Plus comes in a shaker bottle and packets, which are perfect when you're going out to eat. Call 1-800-899-9908, or go to *www.steviaplus.com.*)

PHASE 2: ONGOING FAT FLUSH

You may have these foods in addition to the ones on the phase 1 list.

Friendly Carbohydrates
- Tortillas from Ezekiel 4:9
- Wheat-free, yeast-free bread with sprouted grains and legumes (HealthSeed Spelt from French Meadow Bakery, Ezekiel 4:9 from Rainier and Food for Life, and Sprouted Multigrain from Alvarado Street Bakery)

Vegetables
- Butternut and acorn squash
- Parsnips
- Peas
- Rutabagas
- Sweet potatoes
- Turnips

Herbs, Spices, and All Accompaniments
- Basil (fresh or dried)
- Chinese Five Spice powder
- Dijon mustard
- Mint (fresh or dried)
- Oregano (dried)
- Rosemary (fresh or dried)

PHASE 3:
LIFESTYLE EATING PLAN

You may have these foods in addition to the ones on the phase 1 and phase 2 lists.

Dairy Products
- Cheddar cheese
- Cottage cheese, low-fat or 2% (Friendship, Old Home)
- Cream
- Cream cheese
- Goat cheese
- Grated Parmesan cheese (occasionally)
- Mozzarella cheese
- Nonfat, low-fat, or whole milk yogurt
- Parmesan cheese
- Ricotta cheese (Calabro)
- Romano cheese
- Sour cream
- String cheese
- Sweet butter
- Swiss cheese

Protein: Fish
- Frozen fish burgers (Northwest Naturals)

Protein: Poultry

Turkey
- Turkey jerky (Shelton's)

Protein: Meat

Beef
- Beef jerky (Shelton's)

Friendly Carbohydrates

Starchy Vegetables
- Beets

- Chestnuts
- Corn on the cob
- Potatoes

Beans

- Black beans
- Chickpeas
- Kidney beans
- Pinto beans

Cereals and Grains

- Brown rice
- Popcorn
- Steel-cut or old-fashioned rolled oats
- Wheat germ (Kretchmer's), toasted
- Whole-grain pasta

Breads, Crackers, and Chips

- Blue corn chips
- Corn tortillas
- Scandinavian-style crispbreads (Bran-a-Krisp, Kauli, and Wasa)

Fruits

- Grapes
- Pineapples

Nuts and Seeds

- Almond butter
- Almonds
- Caraway seeds
- Filberts
- Macadamia nuts
- Peanut butter
- Peanuts
- Pecans
- Poppy seeds
- Pumpkin seeds
- Sesame butter of Tahina (Arrowhead Mills, Westbrae)
- Sunflower seeds
- Walnuts

Other Products
- Agar-agar (seaweed gelatin)

Herbs, Spices, and All Accompaniments
- Allspice
- Cardamom
- Horseradish
- Marjoram
- Nutmeg
- Saffron
- Sage
- Savory
- Sea salt or mineral-enhanced salt (Celtic Salt, Real Salt, Bioforce, Herbamare Salt, Trocomare Herbal Salt, and Cardia Salt for those who need a higher-potassium salt substitute)
- Tarragon
- Thyme

Condiments
- Angostura bitters
- Capers
- Mayonnaise: Spectrum Naturals organic mayonnaise

Cooking Products and Extras
- Carob powder
- Cocoa powder

Flavor Extracts
- Flavor extracts (vanilla, anise, almond, lemon, lime, mint, rum, orange)
- Sugarless vanilla and chocolate extracts [Nielsen-Massey Sugarless Vanilla Extract, Lochhead Vanilla (314-772-2124), and Star Kay White's Pure Chocolate Extract (*www.atkinscenter.com*)].

Oils, and Sprays
- Avocado
- Extra-virgin and unfiltered olive oils (Kroger, Bertolli, Private Selection, Oligra, Mezzetta, Sasso)

- Olive oil-based sprays
- Rice bran oil (Tsuno)
- Sesame and toasted sesame oils (Spectrum, Eden)

Miscellaneous

- Avocado
- Unsweetened coconut

Baking Powder

- Aluminum-free brands (Royal, Rumford, Price, and Schillings)
- Low-sodium, cereal-free brands (Cellu and Featherweight)

Thickeners

- Arrowroot
- Kudzu

Juices and Other Drinks

- Low-sodium vegetable juices (Low Sodium V-8 Juice, Muir Glen Tomato Juice, Muir Glen 100% Vegetable Juice, and Knudsen Organic Very Veggie Juice)

Acceptable Teas and Coffees

- Decaffeinated green tea
- Fennel tea
- Hibiscus tea (Tazo Om and Green Ginger, The Republic of Tea Moroccan Mint, Celestial Seasonings Green Tea with Antioxidants)
- Peppermint tea
- Red tea (rooibos tea)
- Rosehip tea
- Taheebo (good for yeast control)

PHASE 3:
SPECIAL OCCASION

Fats

- Coconut milk
- Heavy cream
- Whipped cream

Fruits

- Applesauce, unsweetened
- Dates
- Dried apricots
- Dried figs
- Mango
- Papaya
- Prunes or dried plums
- Raisins or currants

Sweeteners

- Blackstrap molasses
- Date sugar (Bob's Red Mill)
- Maple syrup
- Natural, unheated honey
- Unsweetened fruit juice
- Unsweetened fruit preserves

Friendly Carbohydrates

- Almond meal

Flavor Enhancers

- Pernod
- Rum
- Sherry
- Vermouth
- Wheat-free, low-sodium tamari
- Wine (organic and sulfite-free like Frey, Fetzer, Summerhill Estate Winery, Organic Wine Company, Honey Run Winery, Hallcrest Vineyards, and Chinabend Vineyards; available at health food stores and gourmet outlets)

Notes